DOES MY CHILD HAVE A
FOOD ALLERGY?

Jackie Garrett, MD

A note from the author

Food allergy is an unfortunate health event that happens because of an immune response that can be reproduced with each exposure to a particular food. Food allergies affect approximately 6 million children (8% of children) in the United States alone. This may seem like a small number, but for the families who are affected, the path to diagnosis can be long and filled with unnecessary procedures. Food allergies can present themselves in various ways. It is easy to tell that someone is having a food allergic reaction when they have trouble breathing every time they finish eating a particular food. Whereas, it is the subtle manifestations that can be frustrating to diagnose in a timely fashion.

In my day to day practice, I come across families who have had a battery of unnecessary tests to finally reach the correct diagnosis. Others are incorrectly diagnosed with food allergies when they actually have an enzyme deficiency. Some of these children, and their parents, end up malnourished after having their diets restricted. Their parents come in scared that their children cannot eat normally or lead a normal life because they are at risk of a reaction. Others are frustrated because these diets are nearly impossible to maintain.

This book is for those parents. The breastfeeding mom who is told to eliminate 8 foods from her diet, which makes her life torture because she cannot maintain a healthy diet and keep nursing. The mom of 3 children under age 4 with the new baby who has the rash that just will not go away, no matter what new medicine she tries. The dad who is home alone with the baby for the first time and is unsure whether to call the pediatrician because the baby keeps vomiting the formula. This book is a quick guide to help you figure out if your child is experiencing a food allergic reaction.

I have divided this book into chapters by symptom category. With some sections I have included examples, not based on any one patient. They are fictional examples to help you see how subtle food allergic reactions can be initially.

I hope this book helps alleviate parental fears and public confusion about food allergies. I also hope that it helps to guide your discussion with your primary care provider and specialist.

Dr. Jackie Garrett

Contents

Chapter 1 : Rashes

There are three main types of rashes that can be a cause of great concern for parents when they go see an allergist. They are hives, contact dermatitis and atopic dermatitis. The last one is commonly known as eczema.

Section 1: Hives

What are hives:
Hives are a type of rash that can be caused by many things. Hives can be because of an allergic skin reaction to a food. The rash has various appearances, including small to large reddish or pinkish areas with central swelling. They can look like a fluid filled bubble. Hive rashes can also be described as blotches or welts. They can appear in a straight line, merging circles or small bumps that are spread apart.

Hives are often itchy, but in some cases, can burn. Hives can be part of mild allergic reaction, if only a small amount of skin is involved. For example, a few dots on the face. They can also be part of a severe allergic reaction, if the rash is spread all over the body.

When should you consider the possibility of a food allergy:
If your child always develops hives after eating a certain type of food.

This is an example of a child with an EGG allergy.
Day 1- Your child eats a few bites of pancakes and within 30 seconds (some reactions can take up to 2 hours) develops a few blotches on the face.

Day 4- Your child eats a couple of bites of scrambled eggs and again within a few minutes, they again develop hives. This time the hives are on face and neck.

What do you do if your child has hives due to food for first time:

For a hive only rash- a few dots on face, can treat immediately if you have a food allergy action plan for your child and then call your primary care provider (Pediatrician/Family practitioner). If you do not have a food allergy action plan, call your primary care provider's office immediately for further advice.

For a moderate reaction- Hives on face and spreading to neck, can treat immediately if you have a food allergy action plan for your child and then call your primary care provider (Pediatrician/Family practitioner). If you do not have a food allergy action plan, call your primary care provider's office immediately for further advice.

For a severe reaction- hives are spreading and now your child is having breathing problems) **CALL 911** and if you were given a food allergy action plan for your child, use it. If you forgot to **CALL 911** before doing this, **CALL 911 NOW**.

After the reaction is treated and your child is back to normal:
Avoid all foods that contain the food type that caused the reaction. For example, if EGG was the trigger as in the example above, avoid all foods that contain EGG as ingredient. Make an immediate appointment to talk to your primary care provider about a referral to a board-certified allergist & immunologist.

What to expect at an allergist visit:

Skin prick (scratch) testing- test against possible allergen. You get results in 15 minutes. At times, the doctor will order laboratory testing (called "labs"), for specific IgE that corresponds to the problematic protein of the particular food that is causing concern.

Food Allergy Action Plan to help you and other caregivers treat future reactions in your child.

Routine follow-up depending on the age of the child since some food allergies can be outgrown.

Section 2: Eczema

What is eczema:
Eczema, also known as atopic dermatitis, is a skin condition where one develops repeated, red, itchy rashes. They can be flat patches of dry, scaling skin. The skin can also be rough to touch. For darker skin, the areas where the rash develops frequently, may become darker that the rest of the skin.

Skin affected by eczema can be very dry and sensitive to products used in day to day life, including soap, lotion, laundry detergent and fabric softener.

When to consider a food allergy:
- ❖ Key fact: 36% of children with moderate to severe eczema have a food allergy.

    If it seems like your child's skin is never clear despite changing their bath soap, moisturizers that they use and prescribed creams.

    If your child frequently needs high dose topical steroids to help clear the rash and it soon returns as soon as treatment is completed.

    If the eczema is so bad, that your child requires antibiotics for infections of the rash.

    If it seems like they have more rash than normal skin.

    If they are always itching. Sometimes, these kiddos (and parents!) keep waking up in the middle of night with the itching. Some parents report blood on the sheets in the morning because they scratch so hard.

If within a few seconds to a couple of hours of eating a particular food, they seem to get a new eczema patch or an old patch becomes red or their itching worsens.

What to do:
If you are unsure if a food is involved, you can try to stop giving them that particular type of food only for a couple of weeks. Then, add it back in to see if eczema gets worse again.

The following is an example of a child with cow's milk (dairy) allergy.

➤ 4 month old baby who had some patches of eczema on cheeks and back of neck while mom was breastfeeding.

➤ Age 5 months, started on cow's milk formula. Eczema spreads and has now started to affect belly, back and legs.

➤ Age 6 months, started eating yogurt melts and cheese. This baby is now scratching all of the time, not sleeping through the night anymore and seems like their skin is always red with a rash. Pediatrician prescribes topical steroid cream and changes bathing routine. It helps the rash a little but the skin never is clear and baby keeps itching.

➤ Age 8 months, parents talk to a friend with a similar story. They try to take all cow's milk out of the diet. They change formula to soy formula. 1 week later, baby seems to scratch less. 2 weeks later skin looks much better. Then, they give baby a bottle of cow's milk formula again and within a few hours, baby is itching all over again. So parents stop cow's milk again.

Once you have stopped the food in question again, make an immediate appointment to talk your primary care provider (Pediatrician/Family practitioner) about a referral to a board certified allergist & immunologist.

What to expect at an allergist visit:

Skin prick (scratch) testing- test against possible allergen. You get results in 15 minutes. At times, the doctor will order laboratory testing (called "labs"), for specific IgE that corresponds to the problematic protein of the particular food that is causing concern.

Food Allergy Action Plan to help you and other caregivers treat future reactions in your child.

Routine follow-up depending on the age of the child since some food allergies can be outgrown.

Section 3: Contact dermatitis

What is contact dermatitis:
Contact dermatitis can include skin reactions to
fragrances, cleaning products or certain foods. It can
look like a patch of redness along with a rash on the
parts of the skin that come into contact with the
culprit.

In the case of redness only: redness of the skin can be
associated with hives and with eczema. However, with
some foods, a certain type of redness can happen to
the skin. Citrus fruits, onions and garlic can cause a
type of redness that is known as irritant dermatitis.
With this diagnosis, the child can develop redness
only where their skin comes into contact with that
type of food.

This is an example of irritant dermatitis.

> ➢ School aged child develops redness on hands if
> they are peeling the fruit.

> ➢ For babies, redness develops on chin where
> the juices come into contact.

> ❖ Key point: The redness is short lived and not life
> threatening and does not need medications.
> This is **NOT** the same redness that is
> associated with HIVES!

What to do:
Generally, eating the food without touching it will not cause a reaction. The areas of redness will clear without intervention soon after exposure.

HOWEVER, if redness spreads to areas that were **NOT** in contact with the food or redness is worsening, or if **HIVES** begin to develop, call your primary care provider's (Pediatrician or Family practitioner) office **NOW** for advice on what to do.

After you have treated your child (if your primary care provider advised you to give a medication) and your child is back to normal:
Call to make an immediate appointment to talk to your primary care provider (Pediatrician/Family practitioner) about a referral to a board certified allergist & immunologist.

What to expect at an allergist visit:

Contact dermatitis to chemicals is generally diagnosed via patch testing.

With irritant dermatitis caused by food, testing is not always necessary. It depends on what happened to your child specifically.

Chapter 2: Abdominal "belly" problems

Abdominal or belly problems can be another sign of a food allergy. Reactions can include repeated belly pain, vomiting, diarrhea and food refusal.

Section 1: Abdominal "belly" pain

What can belly pain mean:
Belly/abdominal pain, as a result of food allergies, can be seen in various circumstances. This kind of pain can be a part of a specific protein-induced (IgE mediated) food-allergic reaction called anaphylaxis, where you need an emergency action plan and medications including epinephrine autoinjector commonly known as an "Auvi-Q" or "EpiPen."

This pain can also be a type of non IgE mediated food allergy. Diagnoses like food protein induced enterocolitis (FPIES), as well as eosinophilic esophagitis (EoE) and eosinophilic gastroenteritis fall in this category. Other causes of food associated belly pain can be food intolerance or enzyme deficiency.

When to consider a food allergy:
Food allergic reactions can show up as severe abdominal/belly pain within a few seconds to a couple of hours of eating a certain food. Some children can have the belly pain start several hours after eating a food. Reactions can also present with daily belly pain. This pain can be debilitating, but in other cases it may be only slight discomfort.

The following are examples of different types of food allergic reactions:

Peanut allergy that is IgE mediated: 2 year old gets a sip of dad's peanut butter smoothie and develops a few red spots (hives) on chin within 15 minutes but then the hives go away in 30 minutes on their own.

The following week, this same 2 year old is given a slice of bread with a light layer of peanut butter. After eating the slice, 15 minutes later complains of belly pain, then vomits then develops hives on face.

Eosinophilic esophagitis: 13 year old boy starts eating less and complaining of belly pain after he eats. He is able to keep going to school and has otherwise normal activity. After 3 months, he starts complaining that food feels like it is getting stuck so he drinks more and eats less because belly pain is slightly worse. 1 month later, he goes for a regular check-up and he has lost 15 pounds. He is referred to a gastroenterologist and has an endoscopy that shows that he has a lot of eosinophils "allergy cells" in his esophagus, the part of the body that allows you to swallow food.

What to do:
If your child fits any of the examples listed above, get treatment for reaction, avoid the food in question and please make an immediate appointment to talk to your primary care provider (Pediatrician/Family practitioner) about a referral to a board certified allergist & immunologist. Depending on the timing of the belly pain, your child may also need to be evaluated by a board certified gastroenterologist.

What to expect at an allergist visit:

Skin prick (scratch) testing- test against possible allergen. You get results in 15 minutes. At times, the doctor will order laboratory testing (called "labs"), for specific IgE that corresponds to the problematic protein of the particular food that is causing concern.

Directed food patch testing may also be performed, although it is only helpful when positive.

Food Allergy Action Plan to help you and other caregivers treat future reactions in your child.

Routine follow-up depending on the age of the child since some food allergies can be outgrown.

What to expect at a gastroenterologist visit:

Laboratory testing: May be ordered depending on the doctor's suspected cause of the pain.

Stool studies: You may be asked to collect specimens of your child's stool (bowel movements) for analysis.

Endoscopy: May be done. This procedure involves putting the child to sleep and having a small camera look at the inside of the esophagus (swallowing tube), stomach and small intestines.

Colonoscopy: May be done. This procedure involves putting the child to sleep and having a small camera look at the inside of the large intestines/colon.

All of these procedures depend on symptom pattern and severity.

Section 2: Vomiting

What can vomiting mean:
Vomiting is the body's way of removing food or liquid from the stomach. Vomiting can be due to food allergies, infections, anatomical causes and many other diagnoses. Like abdominal/belly pain, vomiting can be seen in various circumstances tied to food allergies. Vomiting because of foods, can be a type of IgE mediated food allergy, non IgE mediated food allergy or food intolerance.

When to consider a food allergy:
Typical food allergic reactions (IgE mediated food allergy) can be seen in cases of vomiting that start within a few seconds to a couple of hours after eating a particular food.

Another type of reaction that is NOT an IgE mediated food allergy is food protein induced enterocolitis (FPIES). Reactions can happen several hours after eating a particular food and can be accompanied with belly pain and then diarrhea. At times, FPIES vomiting episodes are so severe that a child may need hospital care for intravenous (IV) fluid rehydration.

❖ Key point: Some children with food allergic reactions may experience episodes of repeated vomiting, where they stop vomiting after initial reaction, but the vomiting starts back up a few hours later.

The following are some examples of food allergic reactions.

<u>Sesame seed allergy that is IgE mediated</u>:
2 year old gets a bite of dad's hummus and develops a few red spots (hives) on chin within 15 minutes, but then hives go away on their own within 30 minutes.

The following week, this same child is given a slice of bread in the morning, with a light layer of tahini on it. After eating two bites of the bread, the child begins to vomit repeatedly.

<u>Food protein induced enterocolitis (FPIES)</u>:
4 month old boy starts rice cereal. Day 1 takes only a few spoonfuls. 4 hours later, develops vomiting and keeps vomiting. Then 8 hours later develops diarrhea. The next day, he wakes up completely fine. Parents chalk it up to a 24 hour stomach bug.

2 weeks later, they try rice cereal again. Again, he only eats a few spoonfuls. Again 4 hours later develops vomiting but this time it keeps going on. Because it is now evening, the parents take baby to hospital for evaluation and baby receives IV fluids and a medication to stop vomiting. Baby was discharged with diagnosis of stomach bug.

1 week later, they try rice cereal again and he eats half a small bowl. 4 hours later, he develops vomiting but this time he keeps vomiting and he becomes lethargic. The parents take baby to hospital once again for evaluation and the baby receives IV fluids and a medication to stop vomiting. This time however, he is kept in the hospital for 2 days because he keeps vomiting and has also developed diarrhea. Baby was discharged with diagnosis of suspected stomach bug.

On the hospital follow-up, the pediatrician recommends a food allergy evaluation.

What to do:
If your child fits any of the examples listed above, get treatment for the reaction then avoid the food in question and please make an immediate appointment to talk to your primary care provider (Pediatrician/Family practitioner) about a referral to a board certified allergist & immunologist. Depending on the timing of the belly pain, your child may also need to be evaluated by a board certified gastroenterologist.

What to expect at an allergist visit:

Skin prick (scratch) testing- test against possible allergen. You get results in 15 minutes. At times, the doctor will order laboratory testing (called "labs"), for specific IgE that corresponds to the problematic protein of the particular food that is causing concern.

Directed food patch testing may also be performed, although it is only helpful when positive.

Food Allergy Action Plan to help you and other caregivers treat future reactions in your child.

Routine follow-up depending on the age of the child since some food allergies can be outgrown.

What to expect at a gastroenterologist visit:

Laboratory testing: May be ordered depending on the doctor's suspicion of the cause of your child's symptoms.

Stool studies: You may be asked to collect specimens of your child's stool (bowel movements) for analysis.

Endoscopy: May be done. This procedure involves putting the child to sleep and having a small camera look at the inside of the esophagus (swallowing tube), stomach and small intestines.

Colonoscopy: May be done. This procedure involves putting the child to sleep and having a small camera look at the inside of the large intestines/colon.

All of these procedures depend on symptom pattern and severity.

Section 3: Diarrhea

What can diarrhea mean:
Diarrhea is when the body experiences increased loose or watery bowel movements/stools and/or increased number of stools. Like abdominal/belly pain and vomiting, diarrhea can be seen in various circumstances. At times, diarrhea can be tied to food allergies. Diarrhea, because of a food trigger, can be a type of IgE mediated food allergy, non IgE mediated food allergy or food intolerance.

When to consider a food allergy:
Food allergic reactions can present with diarrhea that can start within a few seconds to a couple of hours after eating a particular food. These are IgE mediated food allergic reactions.

Another type of reaction can happen several hours after eating a particular food and can be accompanied with abdominal/belly pain and vomiting. These are non IgE mediated food allergic reactions. At times these types of episodes are so severe that a child may need hospital care for IV fluid rehydration. Some children may even experience episodes of daily diarrhea with no normal stools.

The following are examples of food allergic reactions.

Cow's milk (Dairy) allergy that is IgE mediated:
2 year old gets a sip of dad's smoothie and develops a few red spots (hives) on chin within 15 minutes which then go away in 30 minutes on their own.

The following week, this same child is given a pancake with a light layer of butter. 15 minutes after eating the slice, child complains of belly pain, then vomits, develops diarrhea and becomes pale.

Food protein induced enterocolitis, FPIES:
4 month old girl starts rice cereal. 1st day takes only a few spoonfuls. 4 hours later, develops vomiting and keeps vomiting. 8 hours later baby develops diarrhea. By next day she wakes up completely fine. Parents chalk it up to a stomach bug.

2 weeks later, they try rice cereal again. This time she eats half of a small bowl. Again 4 hours later, she develops vomiting and 8 hours later diarrhea, but this time it keeps going through the night into midday and the baby is becoming listless. She has to go to hospital for evaluation and receives IV fluids for rehydration. Baby is hospitalized for 3 days.

What to do:
If your child fits any of the examples listed above, get treatment for the reaction, then avoid the food in question and please make an immediate appointment to talk to your primary care provider (Pediatrician/Family practitioner) about a referral to a board certified allergist & immunologist. Depending on the timing of the belly pain, your child may also need to be evaluated by a board certified gastroenterologist.

What to expect at an allergist visit:

Skin prick (scratch) testing- test against possible allergen. You get results in 15 minutes. At times, the doctor will order laboratory testing (called "labs"), for specific IgE that corresponds to the problematic protein of the particular food that is causing concern.

Directed food patch testing may also be performed, although it is only helpful when positive.

Food Allergy Action Plan to help you and other caregivers treat future reactions in your child.

Routine follow-up depending on the age of the child since some food allergies can be outgrown.

What to expect at a gastroenterologist visit:

Laboratory testing: May be ordered depending on the doctor's suspicion of the   cause of your child's symptoms.

Stool studies: You may be asked to collect specimens of your child's stool (bowel movements) for analysis.

Endoscopy : May be done. This procedure involves putting the child to sleep and having a small camera look at the inside of the esophagus (swallowing tube), stomach and small intestines.

Colonoscopy: May be done. This procedure involves putting the child to sleep and having a small camera look at the inside of the large intestines/colon.

All of these procedures depend on symptom pattern and severity.

Section 4: Food refusal

What can food refusal mean:
Food refusal is usually a normal toddler behavior. It can vary from day to day, where your child prefers to eat one kind of food. Then one day, that same child will shake their head, spit the food or just sit and stare at the food!

However, sometimes food refusal can be because of a food allergy. Food refusal can be a type of IgE mediated food allergy or non IgE mediated food allergy. You should suspect a food allergy if your child only refuses to eat only one type of food, for example fish.

When to consider a food allergy:
These are examples of food allergic causes of food refusal.

Child with soy allergy that is IgE mediated:
9 month old boy is offered soy yogurt. Baby takes one spoonful, immediately spits it out and refuses to eat anymore.

2 weeks later, parents try a different flavor of soy yogurt with same outcome.

1 month later, mom gives baby a smoothie made with soymilk. He drinks 1 ounce and develops hives all over his body.

Child with Eosinophilic esophagitis (EoE):
8 year old girl who has always been small for her age is refusing to eat very much and she says it is because her belly hurts. She says that the pain is worse when

she eats french fries, mashed potatoes and anything with cow's milk (dairy).

What to do:
If your child has persistent food refusal, then you should make an immediate appointment to talk to your primary care provider (Pediatrician/Family practitioner). If this is ongoing, then your child may be referred to a board certified gastroenterologist and/or allergist & immunologist.

What to expect at an allergist visit:

Skin prick (scratch) testing- test against possible allergen. You get results in 15 minutes. At times, the doctor will order laboratory testing (called "labs"), for specific IgE that corresponds to the problematic protein of the particular food that is causing concern.

Directed food patch testing may also be performed, although it is only helpful when positive.

Food Allergy Action Plan to help you and other caregivers treat future reactions in your child.

Routine follow-up depending on the age of the child since some food allergies can be outgrown.

What to expect at a gastroenterologist visit:

Laboratory testing: May be ordered depending on the doctor's suspicion of the   cause of your child's symptoms.

Stool studies: You may be asked to collect specimens of your child's stool (bowel movements) for analysis.

Endoscopy: May be done. This procedure involves putting the child to sleep and having a small camera look at the inside of the esophagus (swallowing tube), stomach and small intestines.

Colonoscopy: May be done. This procedure involves putting the child to sleep and having a small camera look at the inside of the large intestines/colon.

All of these procedures depend on symptom pattern and severity.

Section 5: Constipation

Constipation is not a form of food allergy. Depending on the age of the child when constipation starts, there can be a variety of causes. Diet is a common cause of constipation, but the current standard skin (prick testing), blood (IgE testing) and patch testing offered by board certified allergists and immunologists cannot be used to identify foods that commonly are associated with constipation.

In older children, there can be acquired causes, including new medical problems where constipation can develop. There are some medical conditions, for example Celiac disease, where certain foods can trigger constipation. However, with these medical conditions, standard food allergy skin testing or food allergy (IgE) blood testing is not helpful and is not indicated.

What to do:
If your child has constipation, then you should make an appointment to talk to your primary care provider (Pediatrician/Family practitioner), about how to treat constipation. If these treatments not helpful and constipation persists, then your child may be referred to a board certified gastroenterologist for further evaluation.

What to expect at a gastroenterologist visit:

Laboratory testing: May be ordered depending on the doctor's suspicion of the cause of your child's symptoms.

Stool studies: You may be asked to collect specimens of your child's stool (bowel movements) for analysis.

Endoscopy: May be done. This procedure involves putting the child to sleep and having a small camera look at the inside of the esophagus (swallowing tube), stomach and small intestines.

Colonoscopy: May be done. This procedure involves putting the child to sleep and having a small camera look at the inside of the large intestines/colon.

All of these procedures depend on symptom pattern and severity.

Chapter 3: Breathing problems

When most people hear that breathing problems can be associated with eating a food, they can figure out that this is a food allergic reaction. However, sometimes in the moment a reasonable person may dismiss small occurrences until they think back on them, or when similar episodes occur at a later time.

Section 1: Sneezing

What can sneezing mean:
Sneezing may due to illness, inhaling an irritant, pollen allergies, animal allergies, and in some cases food allergies.

When to consider food allergy:
If your child always sneezes within a few seconds to 2 hours after eating a particular food, even when they are otherwise well.

This is an example of a food allergic cause for sneezing:

Shellfish allergy:
16 year old goes out to eat. Friends order a shrimp cocktail appetizer. She eats 1 shrimp only and immediately begins sneezing. After 30 minutes sneezing stops. She does not eat any shellfish for a bit.

3 months later, she goes to a clam bake and eats a few coconut shrimp. She immediately starts sneezing, this time it lasts 45 minutes. She feels like her throat is sore with mucous and so she leaves. She feels better by the next day.

1 week later, she eats a few spoonfuls of clam chowder, she begins coughing then she develops hives. She calls her doctor's office for advice on what to do. She calls 911 as she is advised to do and after she leaves the hospital, she schedules a follow-up with her doctor because she is worried she has developed a shellfish allergy.

What to do:
If your child fits the example listed above, then you should get treatment for the reaction, then avoid the food in question and please make an immediate appointment to talk to your primary care provider (Pediatrician or Family practitioner) about a referral to a board certified allergist & immunologist.

What to expect at an allergist visit:

Skin prick (scratch) testing- test against possible allergen. You get results in 15 minutes. At times, the doctor will order laboratory testing (called "labs"), for specific IgE that corresponds to the problematic protein of the particular food that is causing concern.

Food Allergy Action Plan to help you and other caregivers treat future reactions in your child.

Routine follow-up depending on the age of the child since some food allergies can be outgrown.

Section 2: Nasal congestion "aka stuffy nose"

What can nasal congestion mean:
Nasal congestion, commonly known as a stuffy nose, in a child is often due to illness, like a cold. In some cases, it can be due to indoor and outdoor allergens like pollen or animal allergies. In other cases, it can be because of a food allergen.

When to consider food allergy:
If your child always becomes congested within a few minutes to a couple of hours after eating a particular food, even when they are otherwise well.

The following is an example of food allergy to fish.
8 year old goes out to eat with family. Dad orders fish and chips. He tastes a bite of his fish and begins sneezing and feels congested. By next day, it goes away. He does not eat any fish for a bit.

3 months later, they go out to eat again. This time family orders salmon patties as appetizer. He takes a few bites of a patty, becomes extremely congested, then begins coughing then develops hives. Parents take him immediately to emergency room. Doctors and parents are concerned that he has developed a fish allergy.

What to do:
If your child fits the example listed above, then you should get treatment for the reaction, avoid the food

in question, then make an immediate appointment to talk to your primary care provider (Pediatrician or Family practitioner) about a referral to a board certified allergist & immunologist.

What to expect at an allergist visit:

Skin prick (scratch) testing- test against possible allergen. You get results in 15 minutes. At times, the doctor will order laboratory testing (called "labs"), for specific IgE that corresponds to the problematic protein of the particular food that is causing concern.

Food Allergy Action Plan to help you and other caregivers treat future reactions in your child.

Routine follow-up depending on the age of the child since some food allergies can be outgrown.

Section 3: Cough

What can a cough mean:
Coughing is a way that our body helps us to clear our airways. We cough if we inhale a large amount of smoke. We cough if we accidentally choke on a drink or food. We cough when we are sick and need to get the mucous out of our chest. Some of us cough because we are having an allergic reaction.

When to consider food allergy:
If your child always coughs within a few seconds to a couple of hours after eating a particular food, even when they are otherwise well.

This is an example of a child with a walnut allergy:
10 year old eats a mini brownie with crushed walnuts and begins coughing. He drinks water and in an hour cough has stopped.

1 month later, he eats a banana nut muffin. He begins coughing, gasping for air and turns blue. 911 is called and he receives epinephrine and all symptoms go away within 15 minutes. Parents are told by their pediatrician to avoid all tree nuts until he is seen by a board certified allergist and immunologist.

What to do:
If your child fits the example listed above, then you should get treatment for the reaction, then avoid the food in question and please make an appointment to talk to your primary care provider (Pediatrician or Family practitioner) about a referral to a board certified allergist & immunologist.

What to expect at an allergist visit:

Skin prick (scratch) testing- test against possible allergen. You get results in 15 minutes. At times, the doctor will order laboratory testing (called "labs"), for specific IgE that corresponds to the problematic protein of the particular food that is causing concern.

Food Allergy Action Plan to help you and other caregivers treat future reactions in your child.

Routine follow-up depending on the age of the child since some food allergies can be outgrown.

Chapter 5: Other problems

This chapter focuses on other symptoms that parents are worried may be due to food allergies.

Section 1: Poor weight gain or poor growth

What can growth or weight gain problems mean:
Part of the wonder of having children is watching them grow. Growth problems may present as a child who was growing well and is no longer either staying on their weight and/or height curve. Growth problems can also show up in babies or children who have difficulty gaining weight.

At times, these problems also come with food refusal, abdominal/belly pain or even abnormal stools (constipation/diarrhea). Causes can vary from gene defects like cystic fibrosis, autoimmune disorders like thyroid disease or celiac disease, and yes, at times food allergies. This is not a comprehensive list of all possible causes, but the diagnoses that I have mentioned may help as a reference for some diagnoses your child may receive.

When to consider a food allergy:
Some food allergic diagnoses like eosinophilic esophagitis (EoE) and eosinophilic gastroenteritis can cause growth problems or even malnutrition. If your child is also having food refusal, complaints of belly pain or changes in stool, these diagnoses may be considered.

The following are examples of non IgE mediated food allergic causes of growth problems.

Child with eosinophilic esophagitis:
8 year old boy starts eating less and complaining of belly pain after he eats. He is able to keep going to school and has normal activity. After 3 months, he

starts complaining that food feels like it is getting stuck so he drinks more and eats less because belly pain is slightly worse.

6 months later, he goes for a regular check-up and he has lost 10 pounds. The pediatrician orders labs and they are normal. He is then referred to a gastroenterologist and has an endoscopy that shows that he has a lot of eosinophils "allergy cells" in his esophagus, the part of the body that allows you to swallow food.

Child with eosinophilic gastroenteritis:
7 year old girl starts eating less and complaining of belly pain after she eats. After 1 month, she tells her parents that her bowel movements have changed and they are really runny. She is starting to miss school because she has bowel movements multiple times a day.

After 2 weeks she is brought to pediatrician and is tested for infections but everything is normal. She eats less and she has bowel movements less often but she continues with belly pain.
She is then referred to a gastroenterologist because she has lost 10 pounds and has an endoscopy and colonoscopy that shows that he has a lot of eosinophils "allergy cells" in stomach and colon.

What to do if you suspect a food allergy:
Generally, in these cases your primary care provider (Pediatrician or Family practitioner) starts an evaluation with various steps to try at home and if needed, some blood, urine or stool testing. If the evaluation is normal and all of the interventions for the typical causes of childhood growth problems do not work, then you can make an appointment to talk to your primary care provider about a referral to a

board certified gastroenterologist, along with a board certified allergist & immunologist.

What to expect at a gastroenterologist visit:
Laboratory testing: May be ordered depending on the doctor's suspected cause of the pain.

Stool studies: You may be asked to collect specimens of your child's stool (bowel movements) for analysis.

Endoscopy: May be done. This procedure involves putting the child to sleep and having a small camera look at the inside of the esophagus (swallowing tube), stomach and small intestines.

Colonoscopy: May be done. This procedure involves putting the child to sleep and having a small camera look at the inside of the large intestines/colon.

All of these procedures depend on symptom pattern and severity.

What to expect at an allergist visit:
Skin prick (scratch) testing- test against possible allergen. You get results in 15 minutes. At times, the doctor will order laboratory testing (called "labs"), for specific IgE that corresponds to the problematic protein of the particular food that is causing concern. This is often followed by directed food patch testing may also be performed. With patch testing, results are available in 2 to 3 days.

Poor weight gain and poor growth is NOT an IgE mediated food allergy which means that the treatment will not include an emergency food allergy action plan, the use of antihistamines or the use of an epinephrine auto-injector.

Section 2: Hair loss

What can hair loss mean:
Hair loss is not a form of IgE mediated food allergy. There can be many causes for hair loss, including infection, nutritional status, autoimmune diseases or an exaggerated hair shedding onset.

If your child is suffering from hair loss, food allergy testing (IgE skin prick testing or IgE blood testing) is not appropriate and is an unnecessary procedure. Make an appointment to talk to your primary care provider (Pediatrician or Family practitioner) about the appropriate evaluation of hair loss.

Conclusion

The number of children being affected by food allergies is increasing. This book is meant to help a parent identify symptoms of food allergies and have your child evaluated in a safe, appropriate manner. I hope this book is helpful to you.

Worrying about your child's health is normal. If your child does not fit one of the criteria listed in this book, but you remain concerned, talk to your health care provider. Remember, at times in medicine, people develop problems before health care providers can find names for these problems and appropriate treatments. Do not lose heart, we are here to help.

Glossary of allergy terms

Allergen: The thing that one is allergic to and causes an allergic reaction. It can be a food, animal, pollen, chemical or medication.

Allergy testing types:

Skin prick testing: This is also called a scratch or puncture test. It looks for immediate allergic reactions to specific allergens. The skin is scratched with a device containing the allergen and then results are available in 15 minutes. It can be performed on the forearm or back.

IgE blood testing: Commonly known as RAST testing but that instrument of testing is less favored now and there are better ways to measure IgE. The blood test measures the number of IgE antibodies circulating in the body against a specific allergen. For example, shrimp. This test should be done automatically in combination with skin prick testing because certain types of children, particularly those with eczema, can have positive blood IgE to a certain food and NOT BE ALLERGIC TO A FOOD. This test should be interpreted by a board certified allergist and immunologist to make certain that the right diagnosis is give. Results are generally available in 5-7 days.

Food patch testing: Can be used to diagnose non-IgE mediated food allergy. The data on the usefulness of this test is varied. It can be helpful if positive in the diagnosis of non-IgE mediated food allergies but a negative test does not rule out the diagnosis. It consists of putting small amounts of a single food allergen in a chamber/small disk on the back. It is left on for 48-72 hours.

IgG food testing: AVOID THIS TEST AT ALL COST! This type of test is being marketed as a screen for food allergies but that is a lie. In all current respected food allergy studies that look at IgG markers for food, it is actually a marker of increasing TOLERANCE. This means that positive results on this test DOES NOT MEAN that your child is allergic to that food.

IgE mediated food allergy:
The classic food allergy where symptoms occur generally with a few seconds to 2 hours of a food exposure. The exception is an allergic reaction to certain meats that occurs 24 hours after ingestion.

Severe symptoms of IgE mediated food allergic reactions are known as Anaphylaxis.

Treatment includes:
- Avoidance of food allergen
- The use of an epinephrine autoinjector (Auvi-Q or EpiPen) for severe reactions, also known as anaphylaxis.
- Epinephrine can be combined with the use of diphenhydramine (common brand name Benadryl), or the use of Cetirizine (common brand name Zyrtec).
- Antihistamines should NEVER replace the use of epinephrine for the management of a severe/anaphylactic food reaction.

- Other medications types of medications can be used depending on severity of reaction.

Diagnosing IgE mediated food allergy: IgE mediated food allergy is diagnosed through skin prick testing (scratch) to the food that caused symptoms, generally after your child has had a reaction. An exception is the new studies that are suggesting some children should be tested to peanut allergen BEFORE any exposure. Also, since some foods are every similar to one another, if your child reacts to one kind, they may have to be tested to other foods in that category. An example is fish allergy.

Non IgE mediated food allergy

This kind of food allergy is caused by a reaction involving other cells of the immune system, not IgE antibodies. Some key differences are that these kinds of reactions do NOT appear within a few minutes to a couple of hours after eating the food. They occur several hours after exposure to the food in question. Reactions usually include vomiting and or diarrhea. These children can also have poor weight gain or food refusal.

Specialist Physicians:

Allergy and Immunology: It is important that evaluations for food allergies be performed by a board certified allergist and immunologist.

This kind of specialist is a trained medical professional who has done additional training and research, only in allergy and immunology.

This additional training is typically 2-3 years after general practice training. The training involves understanding how the immune system works and how abnormal function in the immune system can lead to allergy diagnoses. Because of this training, they are held to practice to the standard of care based on current practice parameters on allergic diagnoses, including food allergy.

Gastroenterology: These medical professionals are also board certified and are called gastroenterologists.

This kind of specialist is a trained medical professional who has done additional training and research, typically 2-3 years after general practice training, only in gastroenterology, hepatology and nutrition.

The training involves understanding how the digestive tract and liver functions. They receive training in nutrition. They are also able to perform procedures like endoscopies and colonoscopies.

Because of this training, they are held to practice to the standard of care based on current practice parameters on diseases that affect these parts of the body.